Super Easy Air Fryer Meat Dishes

The Beginner Friendly Air Fryer Guide to Preparing Delicious Meat Dishes

By Donna Thomson

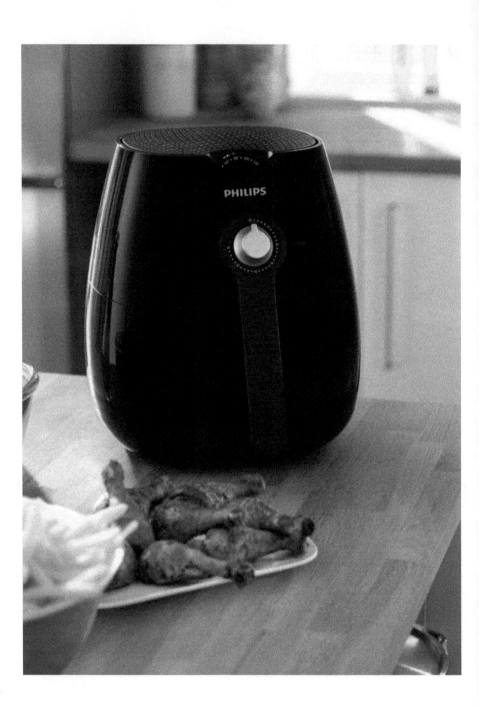

The content within this book has been derived from various sources. Please consult a licensed professional before attempting any techniques outlined in this book.

By reading this document, the reader agrees that under no circumstances is the author responsible for any losses, direct or indirect, which are incurred as a result of the use of information contained within this document, including, but not limited to, — errors, omissions, or inaccuracies.

Table of Contents

8

Ginger-Orange Beef Strips

Servings per Recipe: 3

Cooking Time: 25 minutes

Ingredients:

- 1 ½ pounds stir fry steak slices /675G
- 1 ½ teaspoon sesame oil /7.5ML
- 1 navel oranges, segmented
- 1 tablespoon olive oil /15ML
- 1 tablespoon rice vinegar /15ML
- 1 teaspoon grated ginger /5G
- ·2 scallions, chopped
- 3 cloves of garlic, minced
- 3 tablespoons molasses /45G
- 3 tablespoons soy sauce /22.5ML
- 6 tablespoons cornstarch /90G

Instructions:

1) Preheat mid-air fryer to 330° F or 166°C .
2) Season the steak slices with soy sauce and sprinkle them with cornstarch.
3) Place in the air fryer basket and cook for 25 minutes.

4) Meanwhile, place a pan over medium flame, add oil and allow to warm

5) Sauté the garlic and ginger until wither

6) Stir in the oranges, molasses, and rice vinegar. Season with salt and pepper to taste.

7) Once the meat is cooked, place inside the pan and stir to coat the sauce.

8) Drizzle with sesame oil and garnish with scallions.

Nutrition information:

- Calories per serving: 306
- Carbs: 43.6g
- Protein: 9.4g
- Fat: 10.4g

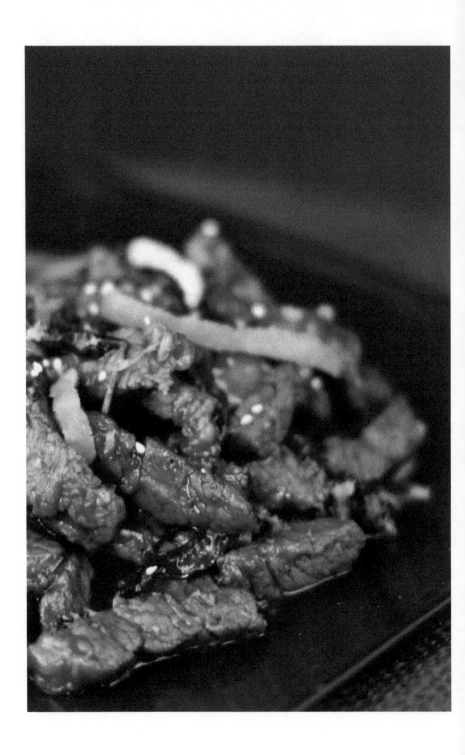

Gravy Smothered Country Fried Steak

Servings per Recipe: 2

Cooking Time: 25 minutes

Ingredients:

- 1 cup flour /130G
- 1 cup panko bread crumbs /130G
- 1 teaspoon garlic powder /5G
- 1 teaspoon onion powder /5G
- 2 cups milk /500ML
- 2 tablespoons flour /30G
- 3 eggs, beaten
- 6 ounces ground sausage meat /180G
- 6 ounces sirloin steak, pounded thin /180G
- Salt and pepper to taste

Instructions:

1) Preheat mid-air fryer to 330° F or 166°C .
2) Season the steak with salt and pepper to taste.
3) Dip the steak in egg and dredge in flour mixture (consists of flour, bread crumbs, onion powder, and garlic powder).
4) Place in the air fryer and cook for 25 minutes.

5) Meanwhile, place the sausage meat in a saucepan and allow it to release fat. Stir in flour to create a roux and add milk. Season with salt and pepper to taste. Keep stirring before the sauce thickens.

6) Serve the steak with milk gravy

Nutrition information:

- Calories per serving: 1048
- Carbs: 88.1g
- Protein:64.2 g
- Fat: 48.7g

Grilled Beef with Grated Daikon Radish

Servings per Recipe: 2

Cooking Time: 40 minutes

Ingredients:

- ¼ cup grated daikon radish /32.5ɢ
- ½ cup rice wine vinegar /125ᴍʟ
- ½ cup soy sauce /125ᴍʟ
- 1 tablespoon olive oil /15ᴍʟ
- 2 strip steaks
- Salt and pepper to taste

Instructions:

1) Preheat mid-air fryer to 390° F or 199°C .
2) Place the grill pan in the air fryer.
3) Season the steak with salt and pepper.
4) Brush with oil.
5) Grill for 20 Minutes per piece and turn the beef after 10 minutes.
6) Prepare the dipping sauce by combining the soy sauce and vinegar.
7) Serve the steak using the sauce and daikon radish.

Nutrition information:

- Calories per serving: 510
- Carbs:19.3 g
- Protein: 54g
- Fat: 24g

Grilled Prosciutto-Wrapped Fig

Servings per Recipe: 2

Cooking Time: 8 minutes

Ingredients:

- 2 whole figs, sliced in quarters
- 8 prosciutto slices
- Pepper and salt to taste

Instructions:

1) Wrap a prosciutto slice around one slice of fid after which thread into the skewer. Repeat until all ingredients are used. Place on the skewer rack in the air fryer.

2) Cook at 390° F or 199°C for 8 minutes. cook. Turnover skewer after 4 minutes.

3) Serve and enjoy.

Nutrition Information:

- Calories per Serving: 277
- Carbs: 10.7g
- Protein: 36.0g
- Fat: 10.0g

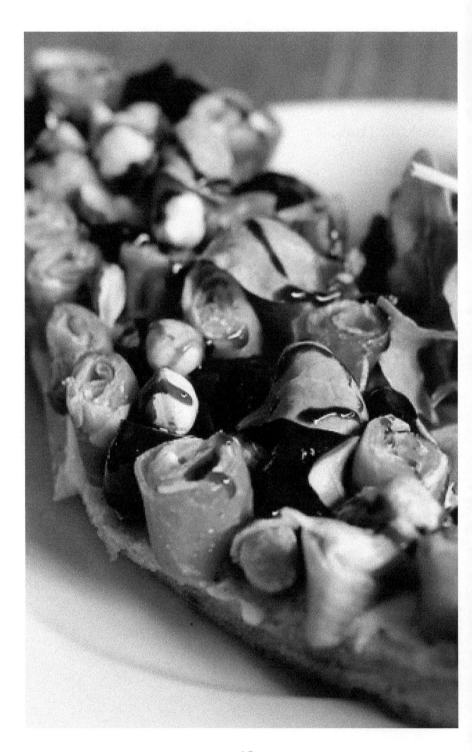

Grilled Sausages with BBQ Sauce

Servings per Recipe: 3

Cooking Time: 30 Minutes

Ingredients:

- ½ cup prepared BBQ sauce /125ML
- 6 sausage links

for Cooking:

1) Preheat the air fryer to 390° F or 199°C .
2) Place the grill pan in the air fryer.
3) Place the sausage links and grill for 30 Minutes.
4) Flip halfway through the cooking time.
5) Before serving brush with prepared BBQ sauce.

Nutrition information:

- Calories per serving: 265
- Carbs: 6.4g
- Protein: 27.7g
- Fat: 14.2g

Grilled Spicy Carne Asada

Servings per Recipe: 2

Cooking Time: 50 minutes

Ingredients:

- 1 chipotle pepper, chopped
- 1 dried ancho chilies, chopped
- 1 tablespoon coriander seeds /15G
- 1 tablespoon cumin /15G
- 1 tablespoon soy sauce /15ML
- 2 slices skirt steak
- 2 tablespoons Asian fish sauce /30ML
- 2 tablespoons brown sugar /30G
- 2 tablespoons of fresh lemon juice /30ML
- 2 tablespoons extra virgin olive oil /30ML
- 3 cloves of garlic, minced

Instructions:

1) Place all ingredients inside a Ziploc bag and marinate within the fridge for 2 hours.
2) Preheat the air fryer to 390° F or 199°C .
3) Place the grill pan in the air fryer.
4) Grill the skirt steak for 20 minutes.
5) Flip the steak every 10 minutes for even grilling.

20

Nutrition information:

- Calories per serving: 697
- Carbs: 10.2g
- Protein:62.7 g
- Fat: 45g

Grilled Steak on Tomato-Olive Salad

Servings per Recipe: 5

Cooking Time: 50 minutes

Ingredients:

- ¼ cup extra virgin olive oil /62.5ML
- ¼ teaspoon cayenne pepper /32.5G
- ½ cup green olives, pitted and sliced /65G
- 1 cup red onion, chopped /130G
- 1 tablespoon oil /15ML
- 1 teaspoon paprika /5G
- 2 ½ pound flank /1125G
- 2 pounds cherry tomatoes, halved /900G
- 2 tablespoons Sherry vinegar /30ML
- Salt and pepper to taste

Instructions:

1) Preheat air fryer to 390° F or 199°C .
2) Place the grill pan in the air fryer.
3) Season the steak with salt, pepper, paprika, and red pepper cayenne. Brush with oil
4) Place the grill pan in the air fryer and cook for 45 to 50 minutes.

5) Meanwhile, prepare the salad by mixing the remaining ingredients.

6) Serve the beef with salad.

Nutrition information:

- Calories per serving: 351
- Carbs: 8g
- Protein: 30g
- Fat: 22g

Grilled Tri-Tip over Beet Salad

Servings per Recipe: 6

Cooking Time: 45 minutes

Ingredients:

- 1 bunch arugula, torn
- 1 bunch scallions, chopped
- 1-pound tri-tip, sliced /450G
- 2 tablespoons essential olive oil /30ML
- 3 beets, peeled and sliced thinly
- 3 tablespoons balsamic vinegar /45ML
- Salt and pepper to taste

Instructions:

1) Preheat air fryer to 390° F or 199°C .
2) Place the grill pan in the air fryer.
3) Season the tri-tip with salt and pepper. Drizzle with oil.
4) Grill for 15 minutes per batch.
5) Meanwhile, prepare the salad by mixing the remaining ingredients in a salad bowl.
6) Place in the grilled tri-trip and sprinkle with additional balsamic vinegar.

Nutrition information:

- Calories per serving: 221
- Carbs: 20.7g
- Protein: 17.2g
- Fat: 7.7g

Ground Beef on Deep Dish Pizza

Servings per Recipe: 4

Cooking Time: 25 minutes

Ingredients:

- 1 can (10-3/4 ounces) condensed tomato soup, undiluted /322.5ML
- 1 can (8 ounces) mushroom stems and pieces, drained / 240G
- 1 cup shredded part-skim mozzarella cheese /130G
- 1 cup domestic hot water (110°F to 115°F) /250ML
- 1 package (1/4 ounce) active dry yeast /7.5G
- 1 small green pepper, julienned
- 1 teaspoon dried rosemary, crushed /5G
- 1 teaspoon each dried basil, oregano and thyme /5G
- 1 teaspoon salt /5G
- 1 teaspoon sugar /5G
- 1/4 teaspoon garlic powder /1.25G
- 1-pound ground beef, cooked and drained /450G
- 2 tablespoons canola oil /30G
- 2-1/2 cups all-purpose flour /325G

Instructions:

1) Dissolve yeast in hot water, add sugar, salt, oil and 2 cups of flour. Whisk until smooth. Add the remaining flour to form a soft dough. Cover and let it sit for 20 Minutes. Divide into two and store half inside the freezer for future use.

2) Sprinkle a flat surface with flour. Place flour on it and knead into a square. Transfer into a greased air fryer baking pan. Sprinkle with beef.

3) Mix the seasonings and soup well inside a small bowl and pour over beef.

4) Sprinkle the top with mushrooms and green pepper. Top with cheese.

5) Cover the pan with foil.

6) Cook on 390° F or 199°C for 15 minutes,

7) Remove foil, cook for another 10 minutes or until cheese is melted.

8) Serve and enjoy.

Nutrition Information:

- Calories per Serving: 362
- Carbs: 39.0g
- Protein: 20.0g
- Fat: 14.0g

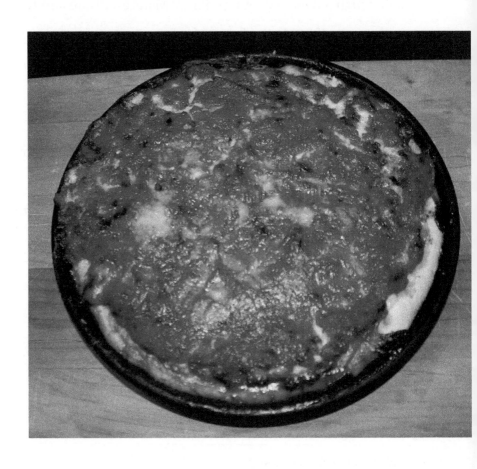

Ground Beef, Rice 'n Cabbage Casserole

Servings per Recipe: 6

Cooking Time: 50 minutes

Ingredients:

- 1-pound ground beef /450G
- 1 (14 ounces) can beef broth /420ML
- 1/2 cup chopped onion /65G
- 1/2 (29 ounces) can tomato sauce /870ML
- 1/2 cup uncooked white rice /65G
- 1/2 teaspoon salt /2.5G
- 1-3/4 pounds chopped cabbage /787.5G

Instructions:

1) Grease baking pan of air fryer lightly with cooking spray. Add beef and cook for 10 minutes at 360° F. stir and crumble the beef halfway through cooking time.

2) Whisk salt, rice, cabbage, onion, and tomato sauce in a bowl. Add meat and mix well. Pour in the broth.

3) Cover the pan with foil.

4) Cook for 25 minutes at 330° F or 166°C , uncover, mix and cook for another 15 minutes.

5) Serve and enjoy

Nutrition Information:

- Calories per Serving: 356
- Carbs: 25.5g
- Protein: 17.1g
- Fat: 20.6g

Hanger Steak in Mole Rub

Servings per Recipe: 2

Cooking Time: an hour

Ingredients:

- 1 tablespoon ground black pepper /15G
- 2 hanger steaks
- 2 tablespoons coriander seeds /30G
- 2 tablespoons ground coffee /30G
- 2 tablespoons olive oil /30ML
- 2 tablespoons salt /30G
- 4 teaspoons unsweetened powdered cocoa /20G
- 4 teaspoons brown sugar /20G

Instructions:

1) Preheat the air fryer to 390° F or 199°C .
2) Place the grill pan in the air fryer.
3) Combine the coriander seeds, ground coffee, salt, brown sugar, hot chocolate mix, and black pepper in a bowl and mix well.
4) Rub the spice mixture lavishly on the steaks and brush with oil.
5) Grill for 30 Minutes and ensure to turn over the meat every 10 minutes after only grilling and cook in batches.

Nutrition information:

- Calories per serving: 680
- Carbs: 16g
- Protein:48 g
- Fat: 47g

Hickory Smoked Beef Jerky

Servings per Recipe: 2

Cooking Time: an hour

Ingredients:

- ¼ cup Worcestershire sauce /62.5ML
- ½ cup brown sugar /65G
- ½ cup soy sauce /125ML
- ½ teaspoon black pepper /2.5G
- ½ teaspoon smoked paprika /2.5G
- 1 tablespoon chili pepper sauce /15ML
- 1 tablespoon liquid smoke, hickory /15ML
- 1 teaspoon garlic powder /5G
- 1 teaspoon onion powder /5G
- 1-pound ground beef, sliced thinly /450G

Instructions:

1) Add all ingredients inside a mixing bowl or Ziploc bag.
2) Marinate in the fridge overnight.
3) Preheat air fryer to 330° F or 166°C .
4) Place the beef slices on the double layer rack.
5) Cook for an hour until beef is dry.

Nutrition information:

- Calories per serving: 723

- Carbs: 79.8g
- Protein: 55.6g
- Fat: 20.2g

Italian Beef Roast

Serves: 10

Cooking Time: 3 hours

Ingredients:

- ¼ teaspoon black pepper /1.25G
- ½ cup water /125ML
- ½ teaspoon thyme /2.5G
- 1 onion, sliced thinly
- 1 teaspoon basil /5G
- 1 teaspoon salt /5G
- 2 ½ pounds beef round roast /1125G
- 4 tablespoons extra virgin olive oil /60ML

Instructions:

1) Place all ingredients in the baking dish so that it covers the surface of the dish.
2) Place the baking dish in the air fryer. Close.
3) Cook for 3 hours at 400° F or 205°C .

Nutrition information:

- Calories per serving: 282
- Carbohydrates: 0.2g
- Protein: 23.6g
- Fat: 20.7g

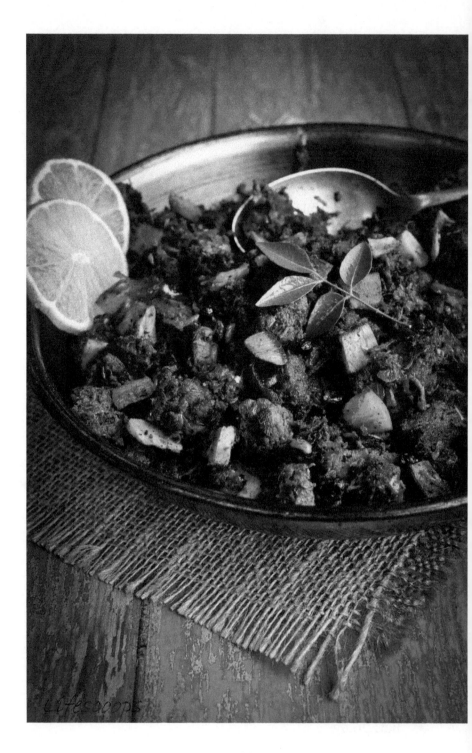

36

Italian Sausage & Tomato Egg Bake

Servings per Recipe: 1

Cooking Time: 16 minutes

Ingredients:

- ½ Italian sausage, sliced into ¼-inch thick
- 1 tablespoon extra-virgin olive oil /15ML
- 3 eggs
- 4 cherry tomatoes (by 50 %)
- Chopped parsley
- Grano Padano cheese (or parmesan)
- Salt/Pepper

Instructions:

1) Grease baking pan of air fryer lightly with cooking spray.
2) Add Italian sausage and cook for 5 minutes at 360° F or 183°C .
3) Add extra virgin olive oil and cherry tomatoes. Cook for an additional 6 minutes.
4) Meanwhile, whisk eggs, parsley, cheese, salt, and pepper well in the bowl.
5) Remove the basket and chuck the ball mixture slightly. Pour eggs over the mixture.
6) Cook for an additional 5 minutes.
7) Serve and enjoy.

Nutrition Information:

- Calories per Serving: 295
- Carbs: 7.8g
- Protein: 14.4g
- Fat: 22.9g

Keto-Approved Cheeseburger Bake

Servings per Recipe: 4

Cooking Time: 35 minutes

Ingredients:

- 1 clove garlic, minced
- 1/2 cup heavy whipping cream /125ML
- 1/2-pound bacon, cut into small pieces /225G
- 1/4 teaspoon onion powder /1.25G
- 1/4 teaspoon salt /1.25G
- 1/8 teaspoon ground black pepper /0.625G
- 1-pound ground beef /450G
- 4 eggs
- 6-ounce shredded Cheddar cheese, divided /180G

Instructions:

1) Grease baking pan of air fryer lightly with cooking spray. Add beef, onion powder, and garlic. For 10 Minutes, cook at 360° or 183°C . Stir and crush every 5 minutes.
2) Remove excess fat and evenly spread ground beef in the pan. Evenly spread bacon slices on the top. Sprinkle 50% of the cheese ahead.
3) Whisk well pepper, salt, heavy cream, and eggs. Pour over bacon.
4) Sprinkle the remaining cheese and then eggs.

5) Cover the pan with foil and cook for 15 minutes.

6) Remove the foil and cook for the next 10 minutes until the tops are browned and eggs are set.

7) Serve and enjoy.

Nutrition Information:

- Calories per Serving: 454
- Carbs: 1.6g
- Protein: 28.7g
- Fat: 36.9g

Maple 'n Soy Marinated Beef

Servings per Recipe: 4

Cooking Time: 45 minutes

Ingredients:

- 2 pounds sirloin flap steaks, pounded /900G
- 3 tablespoons balsamic vinegar /45ML
- 3 tablespoons maple syrup /45ML
- 3 tablespoons soy sauce /45ML
- 4 cloves of garlic, minced

Instructions:

1) Preheat mid-air fryer to 390° F or 199°C .
2) Place the grill pan in the air fryer.
3) Place the flap steaks in a deep pan and season with soy sauce, balsamic vinegar, and maple syrup, and garlic.
4) Place the grill pan in the air fryer and cook for 15 minutes in batches.

Nutrition information:

- Calories per serving: 331
- Carbs: 9g
- Protein: 31g
- Fat: 19g

Maras Pepper Lamb Kebab Recipe from Turkey

Servings per Recipe: 2

Cooking Time: 15

Ingredients:

- 1-lb lamb meat, cut into 2-inch cubes /450G
- Kosher salt
- Freshly cracked black pepper
- 2 tablespoons Maras pepper, or 2 teaspoons other dried chili powder combined with 1 tablespoon paprika /30G OR 10G+15G
- 1 teaspoon minced garlic /5G
- 2 tablespoons roughly chopped fresh mint /30G
- 1/2 cup extra-virgin essential olive oil, divided /125ML
- 1/2 cup dried apricots, cut into medium dice /65G

Instructions:

1) Add pepper, salt, and 50% of organic olive oil in a bowl. Add lamb and mix well to coat. Thread lamb into 4 skewers.
2) Cook for 5 minutes at 390°F or 199°C to the desired doneness.

3) All mix the remaining oil, mint, garlic, Maras pepper, and apricots in a bowl. Mix well. Add cooked lamb. Season with salt and pepper. Mix well again.

4) Serve and enjoy.

Nutrition Information:

- Calories per Serving: 602
- Carbs: 25.8g
- Protein: 40.3g
- Fat: 37.5g

Meat Balls with Mint Yogurt Dip From Morocco

Servings per Recipe: 2

Cooking Time: 25 minutes

Ingredients:

- ¼ cup bread crumbs /32.5G
- ¼ cup sour cream /62.5ML
- ½ cup Greek yogurt /125ML
- 1 clove of garlic, minced
- 1 egg, beaten
- 1 tablespoon mint, chopped /15G
- 1 teaspoon cayenne /5G
- 1 teaspoon ground coriander /5G
- 1 teaspoon ground cumin /5G
- 1 teaspoon red chili paste /5G
- 1-pound ground beef /450G
- 2 cloves of garlic, minced
- 2 tablespoons flat-leaf parsley, chopped /30G
- 2 tablespoons buttermilk /30ML
- 2 tablespoons honey /30ML
- 2 tablespoons mint
- Salt and pepper to taste

Instructions:

1) Add the ground beef, cumin, coriander, cayenne, red chili paste, minced garlic, parsley, chopped mint, egg, and bread crumbs in a bowl. Season with salt and pepper to taste. Form small balls with your hands. Place in a fridge for about 30 minutes.

2) Preheat the air fryer to 330° F or 166°C .

3) Place the meatballs in a mid-air fryer basket and cook for 25 minutes. Shake the air fryer frequently to allow roasting evenly

4) Now, mix the Greek yogurt, sour cream, buttermilk, mint, garlic, and honey in a very bowl. Season with salt and pepper.

5) Serve the meatballs with the yogurt sauce.

Nutrition information:

- Calories per serving: 779
- Carbs: 28.5g
- Protein: 65g
- Fat: 45g

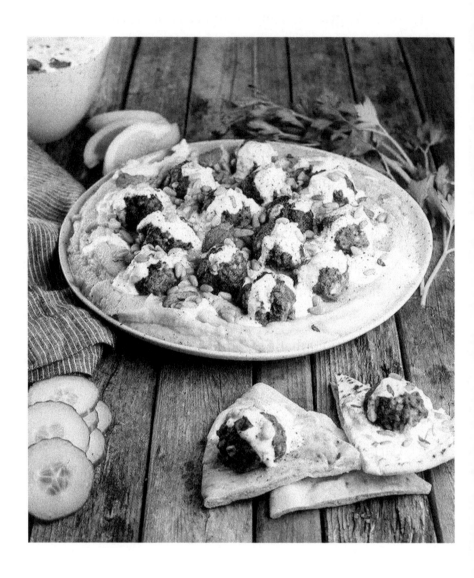

Meatballs 'n Parmesan-Cheddar Pizza

Servings per Recipe: 4

Cooking Time: 15 minutes

Ingredients:

- 1 prebaked 6-inch pizza crust
- 1 teaspoon garlic powder /5G
- 1 teaspoon Italian seasoning /5G
- 4 tbsp grated Parmesan cheese /60G
- 1 small onion, halved and sliced
- 1/2 can (8 ounces) pizza sauce /240G
- 6 frozen fully cooked Italian meatballs (1/2 ounce each), thawed and halved /15G EACH
- 1/2 cup shredded part-skim mozzarella cheese /65G
- 1/2 cup shredded cheddar cheese /65G

Instructions:

1) Grease the baking pan of the air fryer lightly with cooking spray.
2) Spread pizza crust evenly on the pan. Spread sauce on it. Sprinkle with parmesan, Italian seasoning, and garlic powder.
3) Add meatballs and onion to the top. Sprinkle the remaining cheese.

4) For 15 minutes, cook on preheated 390 ° F or 199°C air fryer.

5) Serve and enjoy

Nutrition Information:

- Calories per Serving: 324
- Carbs: 28.0g
- Protein: 17.0g
- Fat: 16.0g

Meatloaf with Sweet-Sour Glaze

Servings per Recipe: 3

Cooking Time: 30 Minutes

Ingredients:

- ½ medium onion, chopped
- ½ Tbsp lightly dried (or fresh chopped) Parsley /7.5G
- 1 Tbsp Worcestershire sauce /15ML
- 1 tsp (or 2 cloves) minced garlic /5G
- 1 tsp dried basil /5G
- 1/3 cup Kellogg's corn flakes crumbs /43G
- 1-2 tsp freshly ground black pepper /2.5G
- 1-2 tsp salt /2.5G
- 1-pound lean ground beef (93% fat-free), raw /450G
- 3 tsp Splenda (or Truvia) brown sugar blend /15G
- 5 Tbsp Heinz reduced-sugar ketchup /75ML
- 8-oz tomato sauce, divided /240ML

Instructions:

1) Lightly grease baking pan of air fryer with cooking spray.
2) Mix 6-oz tomato sauce, garlic, pepper, salt, cornflake crumbs, and onion in a large bowl. Stir in ground beef and mix well with hands.
3) Evenly spread ground beef mixture in pan

4) Place all ingredients in a medium-sized bowl, mix to produce a glaze. Pour the ground beef.

5) Cover the pan with foil.

6) Cook for 15 minutes at 360° F or 183°C . Remove foil and continue cooking for another 10 minutes.

7) Let it cool for 5 minutes.

8) Serve and enjoy

Nutrition Information:

- Calories per Serving: 427
- Carbs: 25.7g
- Protein: 42.5g
- Fat: 17.1

Meaty Pasta Bake from your Southwest

Servings per Recipe: 6

Cooking Time: 45 minutes

Ingredients:

- 1 can (14-1/2 ounces each or 435G) diced tomatoes, undrained
- 1 cup shredded Monterey Jack cheese /130G
- 1 cup uncooked elbow macaroni, cooked according to manufacturer's instructions /130G
- 1 jalapeno pepper, seeded and chopped
- 1 large onion, chopped
- 1 teaspoon chili powder /5G
- 1 teaspoons salt /5G
- 1/2 can (16 ounces) kidney beans, rinsed and drained /480G
- 1/2 can (4 ounces) chopped green chilies, drained /120G
- 1/2 can (6 ounces) tomato paste /180G
- 1/2 teaspoon ground cumin /2.5G
- 1/2 teaspoon pepper /2.5G
- 1-pound ground beef /450G
- 2 garlic cloves, minced

Instructions:

1) Lightly grease baking pan of air fryer with cooking spray. Add ground beef, onion, and garlic. For 10, cook on 360° F or 183°C. Stir and ground the beef.

2) Mix in diced tomatoes, kidney beans, tomato paste, green chilies, salt, chili powder, cumin, and pepper. Mix well. Cook for 10 Minutes.

3) Stir in macaroni and mix well. Top with jalapenos and cheese.

4) Cover the pan with foil.

5) Cook for 15 minutes at 390° F or 199°C , remove foil and continue cooking for the next 10 minutes until tops are lightly browned.

6) Serve and enjoy

Nutrition Information:

- Calories per Serving: 323
- Carbs: 23.0g
- Protein: 24.0g
- Fat: 15.0g

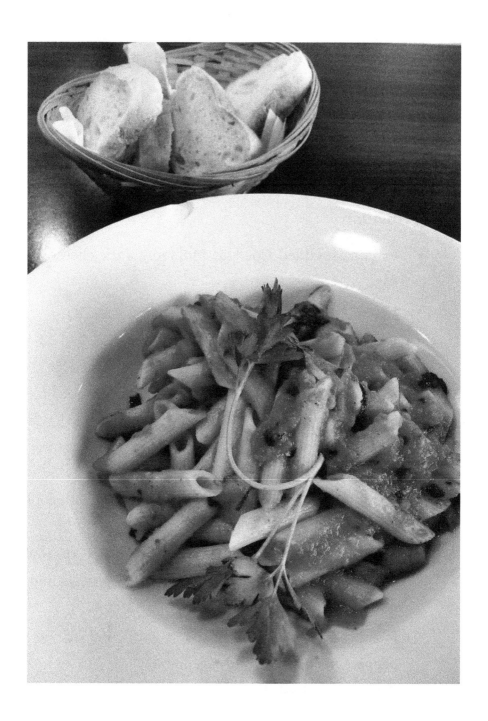

Monterey Jack 'n Sausage Brekky Casserole

Servings per Recipe: 2

Cooking Time: 20 Minutes

Ingredients:

- ½ cup shredded Cheddar-Monterey Jack cheese blend /65G
- 1 green onion, chopped
- 1 pinch cayenne
- 1/4-lb breakfast sausage /112.5G
- 2 tbsp red bell pepper, diced /30G
- 4 eggs

Instructions:

1) Spray the baking pan of the air fryer lightly with cooking spray.
2) Add sausage for 8 minutes, cook at 390° F or 199°C . After 4 minutes of cooking, add crumble sausage and stir well.
3) Meanwhile, whisk eggs inside a bowl and stir in bell pepper, green onion, and cayenne.
4) Remove the basket and chuck the ball mixture a little. Evenly spread cheese and pour eggs on the top.

5) Cook for an additional 12 minutes at 330° F or 166°C or until eggs are going to the desired doneness.
6) Serve to enjoy

Nutrition Information:

- Calories per Serving: 383
- Carbs: 2.9g
- Protein: 31.2g
- Fat: 27.4g

Mustard 'n Italian Dressing on Flank Steak

Servings per Recipe: 3

Cooking Time: 45 minutes

Ingredients:

- ½ cup yellow mustard /65G
- ½ teaspoon black pepper /2.5G
- 1 ¼ pounds beef flank steak /562.5G
- 1 cup Italian salad dressing /130G
- Salt to taste

Instructions:

1) Place all ingredients in a Ziploc bag and allow to marinate in the fridge for around a couple of hours.
2) Preheat the air fryer to 390°F or 199°C .
3) Place the grill pan in the air fryer.
4) Grill for 15 minutes per batch, turnover every 7 minutes.

Nutrition information:

- Calories per serving: 576
- Carbs: 3.1g
- Protein:35 g
- Fat: 47g

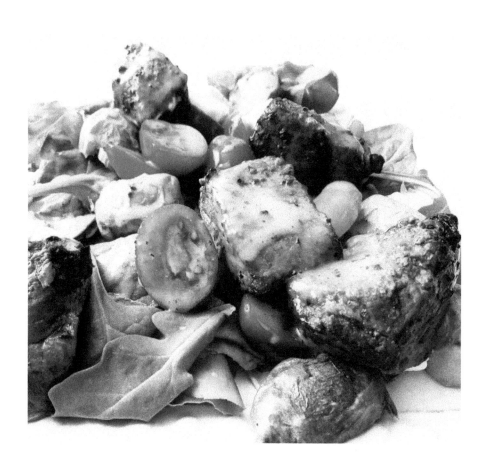

Mustard 'n Pepper Roast Beef

Serves: 9

Cooking Time: 1 hour and 30 Minutes

Ingredients:

- ¼ cup flat-leaf parsley, chopped /32.5G
- 1 ½ pounds medium shallots, chopped /675G
- 1 boneless rib roast
- 2 tablespoons wholegrain mustard /30G
- 3 tablespoons mixed peppercorns /45G
- 4 medium shallots, chopped
- 4 tablespoons olive oil /60ML
- Salt to taste

Instructions:

1) Preheat the air fryer for 5 minutes.
2) Place all ingredients in the baking dish that may easily fit in a mid-air fryer.
3) Place the dish in the air fryer and cook for one hour and 30 minutes at 325° F or 163°C.

Nutrition information:

- Calories per serving: 451
- Carbohydrates: 15.4g
- Protein: 30.5g

- Fat: 29.7g

New York Steak with Yogurt-Cucumber Sauce

Servings per Recipe: 2

Cooking Time: 50 minutes

Ingredients:

- ½ cup parsley, chopped /65G
- 1 cucumber, seeded and chopped
- 1 cup Greek yogurt /250ML
- 2 New York strip steaks
- 3 tablespoons olive oil /45ML
- Salt and pepper to taste

Instructions:

1) Preheat the air fryer to 390°F or 199°C .
2) Place the grill pan accessory in the mid-air fryer.
3) Season the strip steaks with salt and pepper. Sprinkle with oil.
4) Grill the steak for 20 minutes per batch and ensure to flip the meat every 10 minutes for even grilling.
5) Meanwhile, combine the cucumber, yogurt, and parsley.
6) Serve the beef with all the cucumber yoghurt.

Nutrition information:

- Calories per serving: 460

- Carbs: 5.2g
- Protein: 50.8g
- Fat: 26.3g

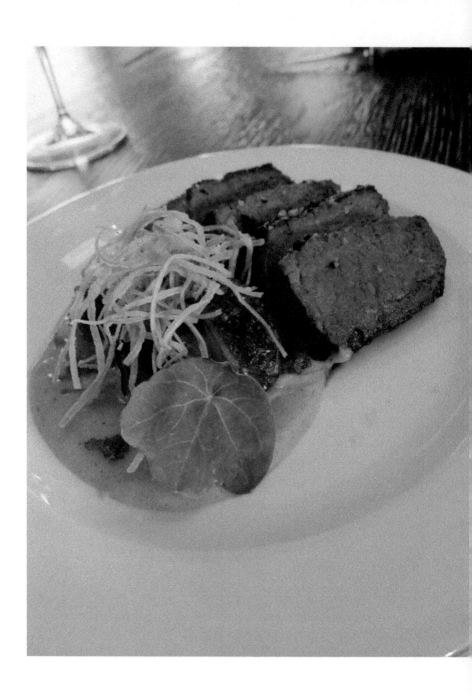

Onion 'n Garlic Rubbed Trip Tip

Servings per Recipe: 4

Cooking Time: 50 minutes

Ingredients:

- ½ cup Burgandy or merlot wine vinegar /65ML
- 1 teaspoon garlic powder /5G
- 1 teaspoon onion powder /5G
- 1-pound beef tri-tip /450G
- 3 avocadoes, seeded and sliced
- 3 tablespoons essential olive oil /45ML

Instructions

1) Place all ingredients apart from the avocado slices in a Ziploc.
2) Place in a fridge allow to marinate for a couple of hours.
3) Preheat the air fryer to 3300F or 166°C .
4) Place the grill pan accessory in the air fryer.
5) Grill the avocado for just two minutes whilst the beef is marinating. Set aside.
6) After two hours, grill the beef for 50 minutes. Flip the beef halfway from the cooking time.
7) Serve the beef with grilled avocadoes

Nutrition information:

- Calories per serving: 515
- Carbs: 8g
- Protein: 33g
- Fat: 39g

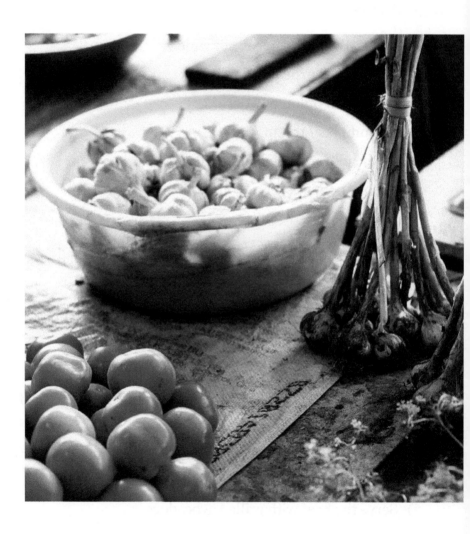

Oregano-Paprika on Breaded Pork

Servings per Recipe: 4

Cooking Time: 30 minutes

Ingredients:

- ¼ cup water 62.5ML
- ¼ teaspoon dry mustard /1.25G
- ½ teaspoon black pepper /2.5G
- ½ teaspoon red pepper cayenne /2.5G
- ½ teaspoon garlic powder /2.5G
- ½ teaspoon salt /2.5G
- 1 cup panko breadcrumbs /130G
- 1 egg, beaten
- 2 teaspoons oregano /10G
- 4 lean pork chops
- 4 teaspoons paprika

Instructions:

1) Preheat the air fryer to 390°F or 199°C .
2) Use paper towels to pat dry the pork chops.
3) Add the egg and water. Then reserve.
4) In another bowl, combine the rest of the ingredients.
5) Dip the pork chops in the egg mixture and dredge within the flour mixture.

6) Place in mid-air fryer basket and cook for 25 to 30 minutes until golden.

Nutrition information:

- Calories per serving: 364
- Carbs: 2.5g
- Protein: 42.9g
- Fat: 20.2g

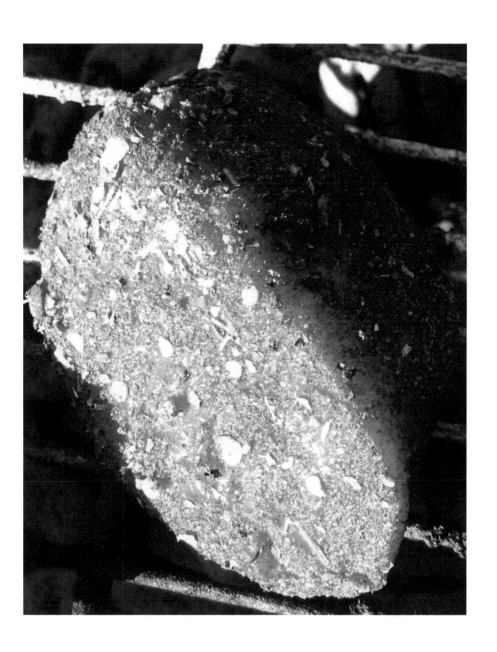

Paprika Beef 'n Bell Peppers Stir Fry

Servings per Recipe: 4

Cooking Time: 40 minutes

Ingredients:

- 1 ¼ pounds beef flank steak, sliced thinly /562.5G
- 1 red bell pepper, julienned
- 1 tablespoon red pepper cayenne /15G
- 1 tablespoon garlic powder /15G
- 1 tablespoon onion powder /15G
- 1 yellow bell pepper, julienned
- 3 tablespoons extra virgin olive oil /45ML
- 3 tablespoons paprika powder /45G
- Salt and pepper to taste

Instructions:

1) Preheat mid-air fryer to 390° F or 199°C .
2) Place the grill pan accessory in the air fryer.
3) Mix all ingredients in a bowl. Coat well.
4) Place this mix on the grill pan and cook for 40 minutes.
5) Make sure to stir every 10 minutes.

Nutrition information:

- Calories per serving: 334
- Carbs: 9.8g

- Protein: 32.5g
- Fat: 18.2g

Peach Puree on Ribeye

Servings per Recipe: 2

Cooking Time: 45 minutes

Ingredients:

- ¼ cup balsamic vinegar /62.5ML
- 1 cup peach puree /250ML
- 1 tablespoon paprika /15G
- 1 teaspoon thyme /5G
- 1-pound T-bone steak /450G
- 2 teaspoons lemon pepper seasoning /10G
- Salt and pepper to taste

Instructions:

1) Place all ingredients inside a Ziploc bag and allow to marinate in the fridge for around 120 minutes.
2) Preheat the air fryer to 390° F or 199°C .
3) Place the grill pan accessory in the air fryer.
4) Grill for 20 minutes and flip the meat halfway with the cooking time.

Nutrition information:

- Calories per serving: 570
- Carbs: 35.7g
- Protein: 47g

- Fat: 26.5g

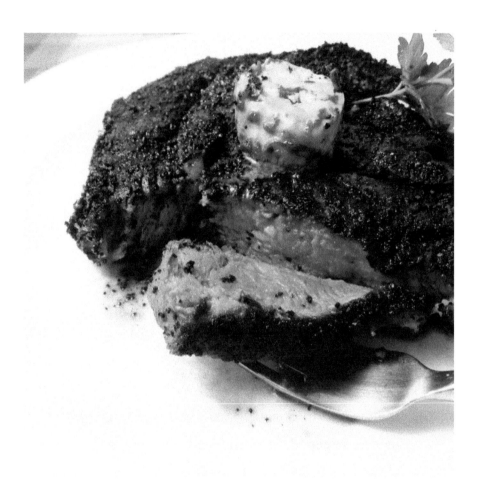

Pickling 'n Jerk Spiced Pork

Servings per Recipe: 3

Cooking Time: 15 minutes

Ingredients:

- ½ cup ready-made jerk sauce /125ML
- 1 cup rum /250ML
- 1 cup water /250ML
- 1-lb pork tenderloin, sliced into 1-inch cubes /450G
- 2 teaspoons pickling spices /10G
- 3 tablespoons brown sugar /45G
- 3 tablespoons each salt /450G
- 4 garlic cloves

Instructions:

1) Boil water in a saucepan, allow to boil, add salt and brown sugar. Add garlic and pickling spices, stir and allow to simmer for 3 minutes. Remove from heat and stir in the rum.

2) Pour the sauce into a shallow dish. Add the pork tenderloin, stir and allow to marinate in the refrigerator for 3 hours.

3) Skewer the pork pieces. Baste with the marinade. Place the skewer on the skewer rack in the air fryer.

4) Cook at 360° F or 183°C for 12 minutes. Turnover skewers and baste with sauce after 6 minutes. If need be, cook in batches.

5) Serve and enjoy.

Nutrition Information:

- Calories per Serving: 295
- Carbs: 19.9g
- Protein: 41.0g
- Fat: 5.7g

Pineapple, Mushrooms & Beef Kebabs

Servings per Recipe: 4

Cooking Time: 20 Minutes

Ingredients:

- 2 tablespoons soy sauce /30ML
- 1 green peppers, cut into 2-inch pieces
- 1 cup cherry tomatoes /130G
- 1 1/2 tablespoons light brown sugar /22.5G
- 1 1/2 tablespoon distilled white wine vinegar /22.5ML
- 1-pound beef sirloin steak, cut into 1 1/2-inch cube /450G
- 1/2 fresh pineapple - peeled, cored and cubed
- 1/4 teaspoon garlic powder /1.25G
- 1/4 teaspoon seasoned salt /1.25G
- 1/4 teaspoon garlic pepper seasoning /1.25G
- 1/4 cup lemon-lime flavored carbonated beverage /62.5ML
- 1/4-pound fresh mushrooms stem removed /112.5G

Instructions:

1) Add lemon-lime flavored carbonated beverage, garlic pepper seasoning, seasoned salt, garlic powder, white wine vinegar, light brown sugar, and soy sauce to a bowl. Mix well. Divide the content of the bowl into 4. Put on part in a bowl for basting. Place remaining 3/4 sauce in a Ziploc bag. Set aside.

2) Add steak to the bag and marinate overnight. Turnover as many times as you can but at least twice.

3) Thread pineapple, tomatoes, mushrooms, green peppers, and steak in skewers. Place on skewer rack on the air fryer. Cook in batches. Baste with reserved sauce.

4) For 10 minutes, cook at 360° F or 183°C . After 5 minutes baste again and turnover skewers.

5) Serve and enjoy

Nutrition Information:

- Calories per Serving: 330
- Carbs: 19.2g
- Protein: 24.0g
- Fat: 17.4g

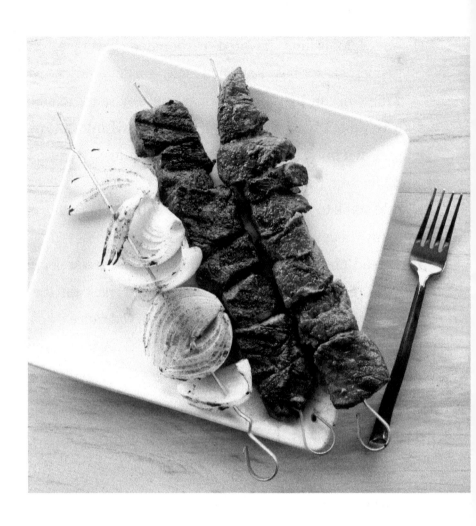

Pineapple-Teriyaki Beef Skewer

Servings per Recipe: 6

Cooking Time: 12 minutes

Ingredients:

- 2 tablespoons pineapple juice (optional) /30ML
- 2 tablespoons water /30ML
- 1 tablespoon vegetable oil /15ML
- 1/4 cup and a couple of tablespoons light brown sugar /62.5G
- 1/4 cup soy sauce /62.5ML
- 1-pound boneless round steak, cut into 1/4-inch slices /450g
- 3/4 large garlic cloves, chopped

Instructions:

1) Put all ingredients except the beef in a Ziploc bag. Mix well. Then add the beef, press the bag to remove excess air, seal. Place in a refrigerator and allow to marinate for a minimum of one day
2) Thread beef into skewers place on a skewer rack in the air fryer. If needed, cook in batches.
3) Cook at 390° F or 199°C for 6 minutes.
4) Serve and enjoy.

Nutrition Information:

- Calories per Serving: 191
- Carbs: 15.2g
- Protein: 15.9g
- Fat: 7.4g

Pork Belly Marinated in Onion-Coconut Cream

Serves: 3

Cooking Time: 25 minutes

Ingredients:

- ½ pork belly, sliced to thin strips
- 1 onion, diced
- 1 tablespoon butter /15G
- 4 tablespoons coconut cream /60ML
- Salt and pepper to taste

Instructions:

1) Put all ingredients in a mixing bowl, mix well and allow to marinate in the fridge for 120 minutes.
2) Preheat the air fryer for 5 minutes.
3) Place the pork strips in the air fryer and bake for 25 minutes at 350° F or 177°C .

Nutrition information:

- Calories per serving: 449
- Carbohydrates: 1.9g
- Protein: 19.1g
- Fat: 40.6g

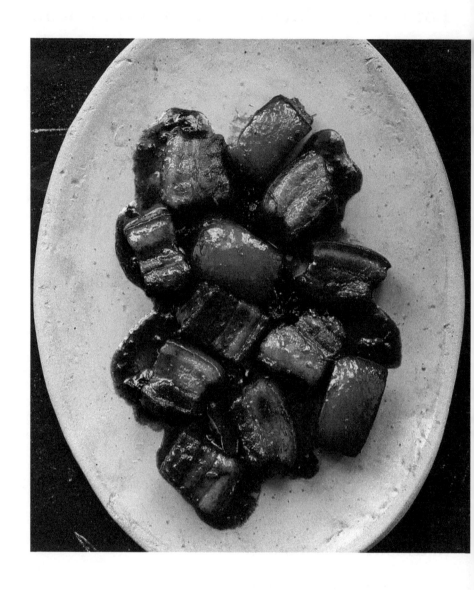

Pork Belly with Sweet-Sour Sauce

Servings per Recipe: 4

Cooking Time: 60 minutes

Ingredients:

- ¼ cup lemon juice /62.5ML
- ½ cup soy sauce /125ML
- 1 bay leaf
- 2 pounds pork belly /900G
- 2 tablespoons hoisin sauce /30ML
- 3 tablespoons brown sugar /45G
- 3-star anise
- Salt and pepper to taste

Instructions:

1) Place all ingredients inside a Ziploc bag and allow to marinate in the fridge for around 2 hours.
2) Preheat the air fryer to 390° F or 199°C .
3) Place the grill pan accessory in the air fryer.
4) Grill the pork for at least 20 minutes per batch.
5) Make sure to turn over the pork every 10 Minutes.
6) Chop the pork before serving and garnish it with green onions.

Nutrition information:

- Calories per serving: 1301
- Carbs: 15.5g
- Protein:24 g
- Fat: 126.4g

Pork Chops Crusted in Parmesan-Paprika

Servings per Recipe: 6

Cooking Time: 35 minutes

Ingredients%

- ¼ teaspoon pepper /1.25ɢ
- ½ teaspoon chili powder /2.5ɢ
- ½ teaspoon onion powder /2.5ɢ
- ½ teaspoon salt /2.5ɢ
- 1 cup pork rind crumbs /130ɢ
- 1 teaspoon smoked paprika /5ɢ
- 2 large eggs, beaten
- 3 tablespoons mozzarella dairy product /45ɢ
- ·6 thick pork chops

Instructions:

1) Season the pork chops with salt, pepper, paprika, onion, and chili powder. Allow to marinate in the fridge for about 3 hours.
2) Mix the pork rind and mozzarella.
3) Preheat the air fryer to 390° F or 199°C.
4) Dip the pork in the beaten egg before dredging inside the pork rind crumb mixture.

5) Place in the air fryer basket and cook for 30 to 35 minutes.

Nutrition information:

- Calories per serving: 316
- Carbs: 1.2g
- Protein: 26.9g
- Fat: 22.6g

Pork Chops Marinate in Honey-Mustard

Servings per Recipe: 4

Cooking Time: 25 minutes

Ingredients:

- 2 tablespoons honey /30ML
- 2 tablespoons minced garlic /30G
- 4 pork chops
- 4 tablespoons mustard /60G
- Salt and pepper to taste

Instructions

1) Preheat the air fryer to 330° F or 166°C .
2) Use all ingredients to season the pork chops.
3) Place inside the air fryer basket.
4) Cook for 20 to 25 minutes until golden.

Nutrition information:

- Calories per serving: 376
- Carbs: 12.3g
- Protein: 41.3g
- Fat: 17.9g

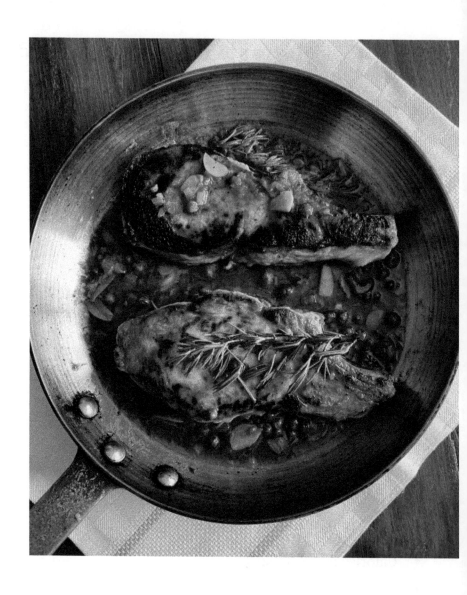

Pork Chops On the Grill Simple Recipe

Servings per Recipe: 6

Cooking Time: 50 minutes

Ingredients:

- 1 cup salt /130G
- 1 cup sugar /130G
- 6 pork chops
- 8 cups of water /2Liter

Instructions:

1) Soak the pork chops inside brine solution, place in a fridge and all to soak well for 2 days.
2) Preheat the air fryer to 390° F or 199°C .
3) Place the grill pan accessory in the air fryer.
4) Spread the meat in the grill pan and cook for 50 minutes, turn over every 10 minutes until evenly cooked.

Nutrition information:

- Calories per serving: 384
- Carbs:16.6 g
- Protein: 40.2g
- Fat: 17.4g

Pork Stuffed with Gouda 'n Horseradish

Servings per Recipe: 2

Cooking Time: 15

Ingredients:

- 1/4 teaspoon salt /1.25G
- 1/8 teaspoon pepper /0.625G
- 2 cups fresh baby spinach /260G
- 2 pork sirloin cutlets (3 ounces or 90G each)
- 2 slices smoked Gouda cheese (about 2 ounces)
- 2 tablespoons grated Parmesan cheese /30G
- 2 tablespoons horseradish mustard /30G
- 3 tablespoons dry bread crumbs /45G

Instructions:

1) Mix well Parmesan and bread crumbs.
2) Season pork with pepper and salt. Add spinach and cheese on each cutlet and fold to enclose filling. Secure the pork with a tooth pig
3) Brush mustard on the pork and dip in crumb mixture.
4) Use cooking spray to lightly grease the baking pan of the air fryer. Add pork.
5) For 15 minutes, cook at 330° F or 166°C . turn the pork over halfway through cooking.
6) Serve and enjoy

Nutrition Information:

- Calories per Serving: 304
- Carbs: 10.0g
- Protein: 30.0g
- Fat: 16.0g

Pork with Balsamic-Raspberry Jam

Servings per Recipe: 4

Cooking Time: 30 Minutes

Ingredients:

- ¼ cup all-purpose flour /32.5G
- ¼ cup milk /62.5ML
- 1 cup chopped pecans /130G
- 1 cup panko breadcrumbs /130G
- 2 large eggs, beaten
- 2 tablespoons raspberry jam /30G
- 2 tablespoons sugar /30G
- 2/3 cup balsamic vinegar / 167ML
- 4 smoked pork chops
- Salt and pepper to taste

Instructions:

1) Preheat the air fryer to 330° F or 166°C .
2) Season pork chops with salt and pepper to taste.
3) Whisk eggs and milk together. Set aside.
4) Coat the pork chops in flour then dip in the egg mixture before dredging inside panko combined with pecans.
5) Place in the air fryer and cook for 30 minutes.
6) Put the remaining ingredients in a saucepan. Season with salt and pepper.

7) DressS the pork chops with all the sauce once cooked.

Nutrition information:

- Calories per serving: 624
- Carbs: 24.6g
- Protein: 45.6g
- Fat: 38.1g

Pureed Onion Marinated Beef

Servings per Recipe: 3

Cooking Time: 45 minutes

Ingredients:

- 1 ½ pounds skirt steak /675G
- 1 large red onion, grated or pureed
- 1 tablespoon vinegar /15ML
- 2 tablespoons brown sugar /30G
- Salt and pepper to taste

Instructions:

1) Place all ingredients in a Ziploc bag and allow to marinate in the fridge for a couple of hours.
2) Preheat the air fryer to 390° F or 199°C .
3) Place the grill pan accessory in the mid-air fryer.
4) Grill for 15 minutes per batch.
5) Flip over every 8 minutes until evenly cooked.

Nutrition information:

- Calories per serving: 512
- Carbs: 6g
- Protein: 60.1g
- Fat: 27.5g

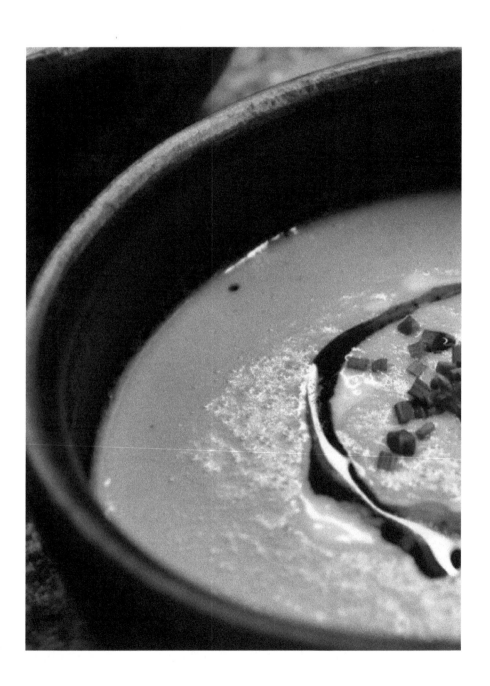

Rib Eye Steak Recipe from Hawaii

Servings per Recipe: 6

Cooking Time: 45 minutes

Ingredients:

- ½ cup soy sauce /125ML
- ½ cup sugar /65G
- 1-inch ginger, grated
- 2 cups pineapple juice /500ML
- 2 teaspoons sesame oil /10ML
- 3 pounds rib-eye steaks /1350G
- 5 tablespoons using apple cider vinegar /75ML

Instructions:

1) Add all ingredients in a Ziploc bag and allow to marinate in the fridge for about 120 minutes.
2) Preheat mid-air fryer to 390° F or 199°C .
3) Place the grill pan accessory in the air fryer.
4) Grill the meat for 15 minutes. Flip every 8 minutes and cook in batches if needed.
5) Meanwhile, pour the marinade inside a saucepan and allow simmer before the sauce thickens.
6) Brush the grilled meat using the sauce before serving.

Nutrition information:

- Calories per serving: 612
- Carbs: 28g
- Protein: 44g
- Fat: 36g

Rib Eye Steak Seasoned with Italian Herb

Servings per Recipe: 4

Cooking Time: 45 minutes

Ingredients

- 1 packet Italian herb mix
- 1 tablespoon olive oil /15ML
- 2 pounds bone-in rib-eye steak /900G
- Salt and pepper to taste

Instructions:

1) Preheat air fryer to 390° F or 199°C .
2) Place the grill pan accessory in the mid-air fryer.
3) Season the steak with salt, pepper, Italian herb mix, and extra virgin olive oil. Cover top with foil.
4) Grill for 45 minutes and flip the steak halfway over the cooking time.

Nutrition information:

- Calories per serving: 481
- Carbs:1.1 g
- Protein: 50.9g
- Fat: 30.3g

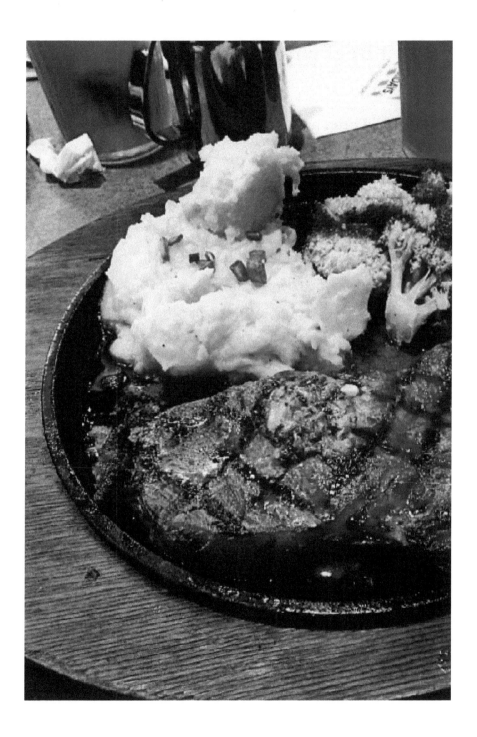

Roast Beef with Balsamic-Honey Sauce

Serves: 10

Cooking Time: a couple of hours

Ingredients:

- ½ cup balsamic vinegar /65ML
- ½ teaspoon red pepper flakes /2.5G
- 1 cup beef organic beef broth /250ML
- 1 tablespoon coconut aminos /15G
- 1 tablespoon honey /15ML
- 1 tablespoon Worcestershire sauce /15ML
- 3 pounds boneless roast beef /1350G
- 4 cloves of garlic, minced
- 4 tablespoons essential olive oil /60ML

Instructions:

1) Fill up the entire bottom of the baking dish with all ingredients.
2) Place in the air fryer. Close.
3) Cook for 120 minutes at 400° F or 205°C .

Nutrition information:

- Calories per serving: 325
- Carbohydrates: 6.9g
- Protein: 36.2g

- Fat: 16.9g

Roast Beef with Buttered Garlic-Celery

Serves: 8

Cooking Time: 60 minutes

Ingredients:

- 1 bulb of garlic, peeled and crushed
- 1 tablespoon butter /15G
- 2 medium onions, chopped
- 2 pounds topside of beef /900G
- 2 sticks of celery, sliced
- 3 tablespoons essential olive oil /45ML
- A couple of fresh herbs of your choice
- Salt and pepper to taste

Instructions:

1) Preheat mid-air fryer for 5 minutes.
2) Put all of the ingredients in a baking dish and stir properly.
3) Place the dish in a mid-air fryer and bake for one hour at 350° F or 177°C .

Nutrition information:

- Calories per serving: 243
- Carbohydrates: 3.1g
- Protein: 16.7g

- Fat: 18.2g

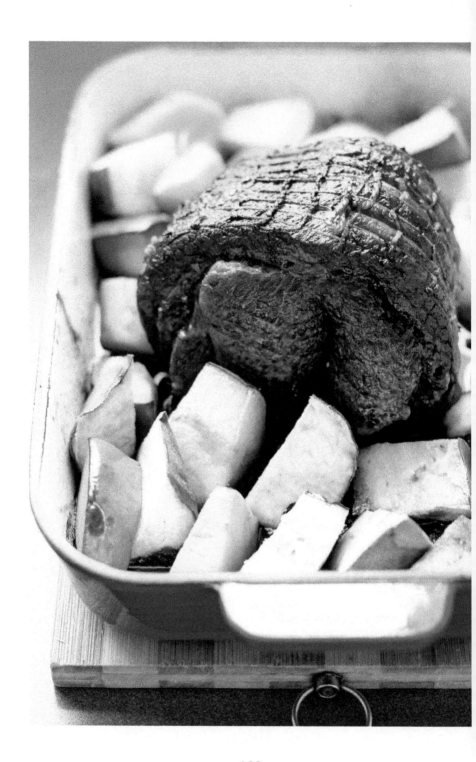

Roasted Ribeye Steak with Rum

Servings per Recipe: 4

Cooking Time: 50 minutes

Ingredients:

- ½ cup rum /125ML
- 2 pounds bone-in ribeye steak /900G
- 2 tablespoons extra virgin olive oil /30ML
- Salt and black pepper to taste

Instructions:

1) Place all ingredients in a Ziploc bag and allow to marinate in the fridge for about an hour.
2) Preheat mid-air fryer to 390° F or 199°C .
3) Place the grill pan accessory in the air fryer.
4) Grill for 25 minutes per piece.
5) Flip the meat every 10 minutes.

Nutrition information:

- Calories per serving: 390
- Carbs: 0.1g
- Protein: 48.9g
- Fat: 21.5g

Saffron Spiced Rack of Lamb

Servings per Recipe: 4

Cooking Time: one hour and 10 minutes

Ingredients:

- ½ teaspoon crumbled saffron threads /2.5G
- 1 cup plain Greek yogurt /250ML
- 1 teaspoon lemon zest /5G
- 2 cloves of garlic, minced
- 2 racks of lamb, rib bones frenched
- 2 tablespoons olive oil /30ML
- Salt and pepper to taste

Instructions:

1) Preheat air fryer to 390° F or 199°C .
2) Place the grill pan accessory in the air fryer.
3) Season the lamb meat with salt and pepper to taste. Set aside.
4) Mix all ingredients in a bowl.
5) Brush the content of the bowl on the lamb.
6) Place on the grill pan and cook for an hour and 10 minutes.

Nutrition information:

- Calories per serving: 1260

- Carbs: 2g
- Protein: 70g
- Fat: 108g

Sage Sausage 'n Chili-Hot Breakfast

Servings per Recipe: 4

Cooking Time: 27 minutes

Ingredients:

- 1 cup freshly grated sweet potato /130G
- 1 cup Mexican blend shredded cheese /130G
- 1 cup sage sausage /130G
- 1 large Anaheim chili peppers, chopped
- 1 stalk scallions, diced
- 2 cups freshly grated white Yukon gold potatoes /260G
- 4 jumbo eggs, boiled, peeled and mashed
- 6 strips of bacon
- Salt to taste

Instructions:

1) Place bacon on the baking pan.
2) Cook at 390° F or 199°C for 5 minutes. Remove bacon.
3) Add sausage and cook for 5 minutes at the same temperature. After 3 minutes of cooking crumble sausage and stir. Continue cooking.
4) Meanwhile crush the bacon.
5) Stir in bacon, shredded Yukon potatoes and sweet potatoes. Return to air fryer and cook for 4 minutes.

6) Meanwhile, Whisk eggs, chilli peppers, and scallions well. Season generously with salt.

7) Remove the basket, mix the mixture well, sprinkle cheese evenly, and pour eggs.

8) Cook for an additional 13 minutes at 330° F or 166°C.

9) Serve and get.

Nutrition Information:

- Calories per Serving: 295
- Carbs: 19.1g
- Protein: 17.7g
- Fat: 17.3g

Salt and Pepper Pork Chinese Style

Servings per Recipe: 4

Cooking Time: 25 minutes

Ingredients:

- ½ teaspoon sea salt /2.5G
- ¾ cup potato starch /88G
- 1 egg white, beaten
- 1 red bell pepper, chopped
- 1 teaspoon Chinese five-spice powder /5G
- 1 teaspoon sesame oil /5ML
- 2 green bell peppers, chopped
- 2 tablespoons toasted sesame seeds /30G
- 4 pork chops

Instructions:

1) Preheat the air fryer to 330° F or 166°C.
2) Season the pork chops with salt and five-spice powder.
3) Dip in egg white and dredge in potato starch.
4) Place in mid-air fryer basket and cook for 25 minutes.
5) Meanwhile, heat oil inside a pan and stir-fry the peppers.
6) Serve the bell peppers on top of pork chops and garnish with sesame seeds.

Nutrition information:

- Calories per serving: 394
- Carbs: 9.3g
- Protein: 43.1g
- Fat: 20.5g

Lightning Source UK Ltd.
Milton Keynes UK
UKHW020815170621
385664UK00001B/147